GOOD STRESS BAD STRESS

RETHINKING STRESS
MANAGEMENT

TIM WATKINS

Waye Forward (Publishing) Ltd
Llanishen
Cardiff
CF14 5FA

ISBN-13: 978-0-9930877-1-4
ISBN-10: 099308771X

CONTENTS

ABOUT THE AUTHOR

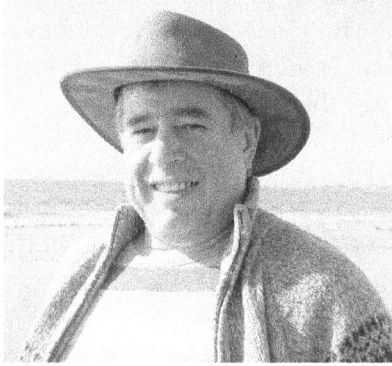

Tim Watkins is a life coach, trainer and a founder-director of Life Surfing, a Cardiff-based community interest company established to help prevent mental illness and to promote wellbeing.

Tim Watkins graduated from the University of Wales College Cardiff with a first class honours economics degree in 1990.

Between 1990 and 1997 he worked as a policy research officer for the Welsh Consumer Council where he researched and wrote a range of policy reports including In Deep Water, an investigation into problems in the aftermath of the North Wales ("Towyn") floods of 1990, and Quality of Life and Quality of Service, an investigation into the promotion of quality of life in residential homes for older people.

Following a severe and enduring episode of depression between 1997 and 2000, Tim Watkins began working for the charity Depression Alliance, running its Wales office, and steering it to becoming an independent charity in its own right in 2005. He continued to run the charity (which re-launched as Journeys in 2007) until 2010. During that time, the Welsh Government appointed him to sit on the Health & Wellbeing Council for Wales and the Burrows-Greenwell Review of Mental Health in Wales. He also played a key role in developing the Healthy Minds at Work project, during which he wrote Taking Control, an audio self-help book for people affected by depression, and oversaw the development of the award-winning Depression Busting self-management programme for people affected by depression.

In October 2010, along with Julia Kaye and Paul Clarke, Tim Watkins formed Life Surfing CIC as a vehicle to address public wellbeing in people experiencing stress or whose life circumstances put them at risk of developing mental illness, and in people experiencing mild/moderate common mental illnesses such as anxiety and depression.

INTRODUCTION

We have been taught to view stress as an illness. Indeed, we have been told that – alongside obesity – stress is the major contemporary public health problem of our age. Where, years ago, public health was concerned with diseases like cholera and typhus, today's experts are troubled by "work-life balance" and the need to improve public wellbeing. They are concerned that stress is the cause of a range of major illnesses including cancers, depression, diabetes and heart disease. They worry that unless something is done, these illnesses will undermine our economy and destroy our public healthcare services.

From this perspective, stress is an enemy to be defeated; something to be avoided where possible. And when it cannot be avoided, it is to be managed and/or treated. The one thing we most certainly should not do is to *embrace* our stress.

But how do we square this desire to avoid or treat stress with the common belief that "some stress is good for you"? This idea came out of the observation of people who succeeded in their chosen fields – artists, musicians, engineers, business leaders, athletes and entrepreneurs. Operating under stress seemed to be a part of what made such people successful. So why does stress seem so positive to them, but so unpleasant and dangerous to the rest of us?

One answer to these questions is that our belief that stress is an illness is wrong. Stress is not an illness – it is an intrinsic part of how we are as human beings. Stress in an evolved mechanism designed to help us cope under pressure, and overcome adversity. Seen in this light, stress is not the enemy. Rather, it is the way we respond to stress and stressful situations that is the real enemy. Our stress response all too often becomes tied up with negative thoughts and emotions around anger, frustration and anxiety. By allowing the experience of stress to be negative, and by responding in an unhealthy and unconscious manner, we make stress our enemy when it should be our friend.

A second answer is that our view of successful people is wrong. What we see of them is the tip of the iceberg; the success at the end of the struggle. Hidden from sight are the years of practice, the failures and setbacks, the learning and the striving that had to be undertaken in order, ultimately, to succeed. The stress involved in this long-term quest for success was associated with positive thoughts and emotions around passion, focus and determination. By making stress their friend, these driven individuals were able to harness its energy to produce positive outcomes.

Seen in this way, we begin to understand why traditional approaches to stress management provide only short-term relief. They are concerned more with relieving and treating the "symptoms" of stress. But without addressing the deeper causes of stress, and without offering a means of utilising the natural biological stress response for positive ends, traditional stress management offers little in the way of long-term help.

In this guide, I want to map out an alternative approach to stress management. Rather than simply providing some short-term stress relief tips, this guide seeks to explore stress in more depth. It examines the underlying social circumstances that give rise to the negative experience that most people think of as "stress". It shows how this negative experience is more often the result of mental and emotional responses concerned with anxiety, anger and worry rather than the stress response itself. It argues that the behaviours that we have learned to use to "manage" this negative stress are often the cause of our long-term problems rather than a solution to them.

This guide offers a range of approaches to stress management from the most immediate emergency stress management through to the long-term process of deploying positive stress to help realise your life's purpose. It offers a range of healthy short-term stress relief techniques that can be used in the place of unhealthy quick fixes. And it provides a holistic approach to building personal resilience in the longer-term.

By viewing stress as a friend to be embraced rather than an enemy to be fought off, I hope to show you that you can turn your stress response into a positive force that will help you to overcome your current circumstances and problems and go on to build a more resilient you; a you who is living the life you always wanted, doing the things that you are good at; the things you enjoy.

"SYMPTOMS" OF STRESS

Technology is the only thing that separates humans today from our ancestors 200,000 years ago. Physically we are more or less the same. Although our brains are "wired·" for the modern environment, our 200,000-year-old ancestors had the same capacity to think and solve problems. The human stress response is also the same today as it was 200,000 years ago. And this is a problem because our environment is radically different. For most of human existence, we were not even at the top of the food chain – that privileged position went to big cats, wolves and bears. From our position in the middle of the food chain, we had to learn how to both fight and flee. If another animal was smaller or weaker, we could hunt it for food. But we had always to be alert and ready to flee from predators that were bigger and stronger than us.

The human edge that allowed us to rise from this unpromising middle rank is that we also developed a brain that included a prefrontal cortex that allows us to think, reflect and problem solve. This allowed us to do things like make tools, weapons and traps. Most importantly it allowed us to plan how we might deploy these technologies. This, in turn, allowed us to overtake the predators at the top of the food chain as our spears,

---

· There is good evidence that neural connections within our brains adapt and evolve in response to our environment and circumstances. This "plasticity" is particularly affected by the things we do and the technology we use to do them. So, for example, parts of the brain that deal with special geography are significantly bigger in taxi drivers. (see Katherine Woollett and Eleanor A. Maguire, *Acquiring "the Knowledge" of London's Layout Drives Structural Brain Change.* Curr Biol. Dec 20, 2011; 21(24-2): 2109–2114.)

arrows and axes proved more deadly than their teeth and claws. And our organised hunting and defence methods proved superior to their strong muscles and sinews.

Our problem today is that our prefrontal cortex did not replace the more unconscious parts of the brain, but simply grew around them. And this means that most of the time we find ourselves flipping between our conscious and rational prefrontal cortex and the unconscious older parts of the brain that do all of our habitual actions (as well as regulating such essential things as heart rate, blood sugar levels, organ function, etc).

This would be okay if we still faced the same challenges today as people did 200,000 years ago. Confronted by a bear or a sabre toothed cat, you would want to be able to respond in the same way. What would happen goes something like this:

One of your senses picks up a change in your environment – perhaps a new sound like the snapping of a twig, or something moving in the corner of your field of vision. Since we are sensitised to change in the environment (this is why you lose awareness of a clock ticking until it stops, or why a car driver can have the common experience of becoming alert and realising they had been driving on automatic pilot for several minutes) our system will send additional energy and focus to our senses to help us become more alert and aware of the potential threat. At this point, many of us experience the hairs rising on the back of our necks.

The information from the alerted senses is fed to an organ at the centre of the brain called the hypothalamus.

It is here that the decision will be made as to whether to switch on the "fight or flight" response. It might be that the movement in the corner of the field of vision turns out just to be leaves blowing in the wind. But if this cannot be confirmed, or if the senses pick up further information suggesting a threat, it might be time to act. Should this be the case, the hypothalamus will activate another organ called the pituitary gland to release a chemical called adrenocorticotrophic hormone (ACTH). ACHT is sent to the kidneys, where it activates the adrenal glands (literally "ad" – on top of – and "renal" – kidneys). These then produce two hormones – Adrenaline (called epinephrine in the USA) which helps the body take *flight* – and Noradrenaline (norepinephrine) which helps the body to *fight*. The adrenal glands also synthesise cortisol, which increases blood pressure and releases energy in the form of sugars and fat into the blood, where they can be broken down and transported to those muscles and organs that need them. The pituitary gland also stimulates the thyroid gland to release thyroxin, which along with cortisol increases the heart and breathing rate.

The main effects of the stress response are:

o Strengthened and energised skeletal muscles (to provide additional power)

o Increased blood sugar levels (the energy supply)

o Increased heart rate (to move the extra energy to where it is needed) o   Some dilated blood vessels (moving extra energy to the parts of the body needed to fight or flee)

o   Some constricted blood vessels (cutting off blood from those parts of the body not required to fight or flee)

o   Enhanced blood clotting (so that wounds can be repaired)

o   Dilated pupils (to increase field of vision)

o   Increased sensory activity (giving the sense of slow motion)

o   Decreased prefrontal cortex activity (to shut down unnecessary thought processes)

o   Perspiration (cooling the body as it burns extra energy)

o   Inhibited digestion and relaxed bladder (shutting down non-essential systems).

Assuming the extra power allows someone to successfully fight off or flee from danger, they will then enter an opposite and equal relaxation response that will involve shaking or shivering and urinating to remove the dead adrenaline and other waste products from the system. They will then rest or even sleep to give the body a chance to repair itself and to allow the brain/memory/mind to incorporate and process the experience (this processing is now thought to be why we evolved dreams).

All of this is fine when you need to run away from a bear (in fact, the aim was not to outrun the predator, but rather to outrun the person next to you!). But most of us live in urban and suburban environments where we almost never encounter predators. Today, people – and their actions – are the biggest cause of stress for most of us. Whether it is dealing with bad drivers on the road, putting up with packed commuter trains, having to listen to the inane babblings of fellow workers or coping with bullying line managers, we seldom find ourselves in circumstances where fighting or fleeing will be particularly useful. If you don't believe me, try it next time your boss is giving you a hard time. Try fighting – just stand up and punch your boss squarely on the nose! I suspect that the momentary satisfaction you might feel will quickly subside when it becomes clear that you are being instantly dismissed and will soon be under arrest.

Okay, if fighting isn't going to work, what about fleeing? Next time the boss gives you a hard time, try just standing up and walking out. What does that get you? You probably won't get arrested. But there is every chance you will be disciplined, and you may even be fired.

You could have a go at freezing. It is common for some animals to freeze and play dead when faced with a threat, so that a predator will think they are dead or diseased and might not be fit for consumption. So you could try freezing next time the boss starts ordering you around. But once again, this could result in disciplinary action for failing to do what you are told.

That's the problem with stress in the modern world. None of our biological responses are appropriate to our social situations. So we just have to suck it up and deal with it later.

The trouble is that just because the thinking part of our brain (usually) retains enough control to remind us that it is a good idea not to fight, flee or freeze, that doesn't stop the rest of our body from running the stress response anyway. When we are forced to suck it up, we are not managing our stress; we are merely retaining enough control not to act on it. Indeed, the evening news bulletins are full of stories about people who were unable to suck it up. All of those stories about road rage, affrays and assaults are essentially stories about people who were unable to stop themselves from acting out their stress response.

Those of us who do manage to "control" our behaviour experience stress in four key ways:

1. Physical sensations, including:

- o   Muscle tension
- o   Headaches
- o   Neck and back pain
- o   Dry mouth
- o   Grinding teeth
- o   Dizziness or feeling faint
- o   Rapid breathing
- o   Increased heart rate
- o   Palpitations
- o   Stomach aches, cramps and butterflies
- o   Indigestion

o Diarrhoea

o Frequent urination (or feeling the urge to urinate)

o Crouched/hunched posture

o Muscle aches.

2. Emotions, including:

o Anxiety

o Anger

o Panic

o Depression.

3. Thoughts, including:

o Needing to be in control

o Worrying about failing to perform

o Frustration

o Pessimism and negativity.

4. Behaviours, including:

o Withdrawal

o Compulsive and habitual behaviours

o Forgetfulness

o Poor performance (e.g. procrastination)

o Disrupted sleep

o Use of quick-fix stress relieving chemicals (such as alcohol, caffeine, nicotine and sugar)

o Use of quick-fix stress relieving behaviours (such as gambling, shopping, compulsive eating and casual sex).

While these unpleasant experiences are manageable if they occur infrequently, they can be a serious problem if the circumstances that caused them are prolonged. Where stress is ongoing and the person affected is unable to process it, the result can often be that they become physically or mentally ill. For example, constantly high blood pressure can result in heart attacks or strokes. Many people will experience panic attacks – which are essentially displaced stress. A panic attack occurs when someone experiences a fight or flight response that has no obvious cause. If there was a cause (either an angry bear or a bullying boss) there would be no panic because the person would be aware of why they were experiencing the stress response. It is only when the response is triggered inappropriately (such as in a supermarket or when queuing for a bus) that panic sets in as the person believes that they are in danger (and becomes even more stressed). Prolonged stress may also develop into a common mental illness such as an anxiety disorder or depression. These occur when the effects of stress become so great that the person affected is no longer able to get on with their lives. While these common mental illnesses are on a continuum with ordinary feelings of anxiety (such as you might have before and exam or a driving test) or sadness (such as you might experience when an event you were looking forward to is cancelled) they are much more profound, and require social support and sometimes medical treatment to get through.

I cannot overstate this – if you have got to the point that your stress is interfering with your ability to get on with your life, the earlier you seek help, the better the chance of overcoming it.

THE SOCIOLOGY OF STRESS

While we tend to think of stress in physical or biological terms, in the Western world very few people face the kind of circumstances that allow for a purely physical explanation. Unless you are extremely unfortunate, you are unlikely to ever come face to face with a large predatory animal. And while some people do get caught up in natural disasters such as earthquakes and floods, these are – thankfully – very rare.

Statistically, the biggest threats that most of us face are of our own (collective) invention. Accidents around the home present the biggest danger, closely followed by road traffic accidents. On top of these, you are at considerable risk if you smoke, drink alcohol or eat processed foods. However, we tend not to consider these to be "stressful". Indeed, drinking, comfort eating and smoking (and for some people risk-taking while driving) are more often thought of as ways of relieving stress.

In the modern world, the things that most people regard as stressful tend not to involve any risk to life or limb. Rather, they tend to be social events and processes that threaten our sense of self and/or our position within society. These events and processes fall into two broad categories: Those involving loss and/or change, and those involving our being stuck in an unpleasant or undesired situation.

Loss and Change

The most obvious loss and change situation is the death of a loved one. Almost all of us go through bereavement at some time in our lives. And it serves to illustrate the way these types of stressor are both events and processes. Most obviously, death is an event. There is a moment when your loved one is alive. But just a moment later they are dead. However, in the case of natural death, there is a process of illness or failing health leading up to the moment of death. In some cases, everyone concerned knows that death is imminent. In others, the certainty of death only becomes apparent at the end of a period of illness. But in both cases, there is a coming to terms with death that begins prior to the death itself. And in all cases – including sudden deaths – there is a period of coming to terms with and moving on from the death. This process will include symbolic events like funerals and wakes. It will include practical processes like registering deaths, sorting out wills and disposing of property. It will also involve the psychological process of bereavement and the sociological process of re-establishing a new social equilibrium in which each person's role adapts to the loss of the loved one.

The process of coming to terms with loss can involve 12 stages:

o *Emotional numbness* – a kind of psychic shock that switches off mental distress in a similar way to the way shock switches off physical pain, allowing you to get through the immediate after-math of loss.

o *Denial* – behaving as if (and sometimes believing) that the person or situation you lost is still around.

o   *Yearning* – having a profound longing for contact with the lost person or situation.

o   *Negotiation* – an internal dialogue with God, a higher being, etc, involving bargaining to restore the former situation.

o   *Agitation/Anger/Sense of injustice* – rage at the situation and the circumstances believed to have caused it.

o   *Helplessness/Hopelessness* – the realisation that things will never be the same again, and the fear that life is at an end.

o   *Depression* – experience of some/most of the symptoms of depression such as sadness, sleep loss, poor memory, inability to concentrate.

o   *Guilt* – both about things that were/weren't said and done to the departed person and about getting on with life.

o   *Bouts of silence/withdrawal* – even as you get on with life, you have periodic lapses

o   *Tearfulness* – becoming overwhelmed by memories or anniversaries of loss.

o   *Self-pity* – about the situation and perceived problems.

o   *Acceptance/Letting go/Moving on* – the final phase of coming to terms with loss in which you incorporate the experience into your wider life experience and are able to let go of the loss and move on with your life.

This process is not limited to the loss of a loved one, but applies to many forms of loss and change, including:

o   Health problems

o   Redundancy or redeployment at work

o   Relationship breakdown

o   Retirement

o   "Empty nest syndrome".

The process may begin before a loss or a change has occurred. Unfortunately, people do also get stuck at different stages. For example, it is common for people to be in denial about a loss or a change even when the evidence for it is plain to see. And the failure to acknowledge and connect with the loss or change can result in feelings of guilt, hopelessness and depression later on. It is usually the awareness that loss or change is going to happen rather than the experience of loss or change that is the most stressful. This is because most people experience a sense of powerlessness in the face of these potentially life changing events.

Knowing that your job is at risk – and with it, the financial basis for your home and family life and any aspirations you might have for the future – is highly stressful. And while being laid-off and having to fall back on an increasingly threadbare welfare safety net is stressful in its own ways, once redundancy becomes a reality, for most people the anticipatory stress disappears as they are forced to take action.

People whose relationships break down often experience a sense of relief when the break-up finally occurs. The stress of strained cohabitation is removed. And while coming to terms with the loss and moving on with life may have its own stresses, once again, it allows for action and re-empowerment.

Stuckness

So even with life stressors that appear to involve loss and/or change, it is the sense of "stuckness" that gives rise to stress. Even in largely pleasant and wished for life changes such as moving home or having a baby, the anticipation of the changes to come gives rise to much more stress than the change itself (which demands action rather than contemplation).

But, of course, too many people find themselves trapped in highly unpleasant circumstances:

- o   The victim of abuse
- o   The girl trafficked into prostitution
- o   The employee who is bullied at work
- o   The person forced to live with antisocial behaviour
- o   The person stuck in a loveless marriage
- o   The child stuck in a dysfunctional family
- o   The family trying to cope with massive debt.

People who experience these types of situation are much more likely to develop mental health problems at a later stage, and are also prone to the whole range of metabolic syndrome illnesses that are associated with excessive stress. However, not everyone – not even most – of the people who experience such circumstances become mentally or physically ill. The deciding factor seems not to be stress itself, but rather, the way people think of stress and the way they act in response to it.

Quick-fixing

Most of us learn responses to stress that appear to help us calm down once the stressful situation has subsided. These can be thought of as "quick-fixes" because they offer short-term relief. However, while they can be useful where stress is transitory, they can be highly dangerous where stress is prolonged and profound.

Faced with stress, many of us turn to one or more of five readily available substances:

o   Alcohol

o   Caffeine

o   Chocolate

o   Nicotine

o   Sugar.

These appear to give relief from the effects of stress by activating the human dopamine system, which causes us to anticipate pleasure (although, unfortunately, they do not in and of themselves give us pleasure). While (with the exception of nicotine from smoking) these are relatively harmless when used occasionally, each can cause serious illness when used in the long-term.

Each of these substances is also addictive. Not only is the stress-relieving property of the substance weakened with use, but we develop cravings for the substance that can be stressful in their own right. For example, the "stress relief" that most smokers claim to experience from a cigarette is only the relief of a craving rather than from any wider stress that they are experiencing at the time.

In addition to these substances, most of us develop habitual behaviours that we use in response to stress. These include:

o   Comfort eating

o   Gambling

o   Risk-taking (e.g. dangerous sports)

o   Excessive shopping

o   Casual sex.

Each of these can give short-term relief to stress. And while they tend not to be damaging to health, they can each seriously undermine social wellbeing. Gamblers can blow their life savings, excessive shoppers can end up in debt, and those who have casual sex may destroy their relationships. And, of course, there are health consequences in the long term. Comfort eaters get fat, and risk metabolic syndrome illnesses. Gamblers and excessive shoppers face poor living conditions. People who have casual sex risk sexually transmitted diseases. And people who take excessive risks may end up disabled or even dead.

Although prolonged and unmitigated stress can result in both mental and physical illnesses, more often than not it is the behaviour that we take in response to stress that is ultimately responsible for illness. The problem is that most of our approaches to occasional short-term stress give rapid relief. So when we are faced with deeper and more prolonged stress, we tend to turn to these quick-fixes in the hope that they will help us to manage. But in the long-term, our quick-fixes serve to undermine our health. And none provide a permanent solution to the causes of our stresses.

Ultimately, the causes of stress cannot be overcome by taking alcohol, caffeine, nicotine or sugar. Nor can they be overcome by taking medications like *Prozac* or *Diazepam*. Ultimately, the only thing you can take to overcome long-term stress is... *ACTION*!

ANXIETY, WORRY, ANGER AND STRESS

People commonly group anxiety, worry and anger together with stress and treat them as if they are the same thing. However, although related, these are quite different phenomena affecting us at different parts of our being. More importantly, they are the most common triggers for our stress response in the modern world. They provide the bridge between unpleasant social circumstances and our biological stress response. As such, they are different from stress itself. And when people talk about "stress management" what they usually mean is "anger management" or "anxiety management" or "worry management". That is, they are talking about the need to manage the underlying thoughts and emotions that trigger the stress response rather than managing stress itself.

Anger is an emotional state that arises in those situations that we commonly think of as triggering stress – those involving being stuck or those involving loss. Consider the phenomenon of "road rage". This manifestation of anger arises because those affected find themselves stuck in an unpleasant situation (congestion) that involves their full attention (to avoid crashes), but where their goal (to get somewhere) is thwarted, and their agency (power to act) is limited. This gives rise to feelings of frustration that can trigger the stress response. This, in turn, can serve to "blind" them to the usual norms of social behaviour, and can lead them to verbally – or even physically – abuse other people.

While we can talk about stress management is this circumstance, we should more correctly talk about "anger management". The very last thing you would want to encourage a driver to do when stuck in traffic is to "relax" in the sense of switching off their stress response. To do so would risk a profound drop in focus (similar to that experienced when intoxicated with alcohol) that could cause a crash. Rather, the aim is to manage the anger so that the stress response is channelled into a positive focus on driving and road safety without the negative loss of control that results in abusing or attacking other people. Stress – in and of itself – is not the problem.

Anxiety is also an emotional response. However, anxiety is always a reaction to things that may or may not happen in *future*. Think, for example, of the last time you had to sit an exam, make an important presentation or take a driving test. The odds are that you struggled to sleep the night before. And the more you told yourself to relax, the harder it seemed to be. All too often in such circumstances, we end up having to perform when we are tired because we did not get sufficient sleep.

Notice that anxiety is not a response to a current event or situation, but the *anticipation* of a future one. Nevertheless, anxiety can trigger a stress response in the present. So, for example, someone who has a phobia (an irrational fear of something such as spiders, mice or the number 13) can become stressed in the present simply by getting anxious about encountering the thing they fear in the future.

So when we talk about stress management in relation to anxiety, we are really talking about learning to understand and manage our emotional response to potential problems that may arise in future.

Worry is a cognitive (mental) process that may concern the past or the future. When combined with the feeling of anxiety about some future event, our minds will often over-think about all of the things that could go wrong. Many people believe this type of worry will somehow prepare them against things that might go wrong. However, more often this type of thinking involves unrealistic "catastrophising" in which the mind engages in often unrealistic or ridiculous scenarios.

Worry and anxiety are intimately linked. It used to be thought that this was a one-way process in which worrying thoughts caused feelings of anxiety. Indeed, this is a central premise of the currently popular Cognitive Behavioural Therapy. However, it turns out that the process actually operates both ways. A feeling of anxiety can arise independently from worry. However, once the feeling of anxiety develops, the mind will often find things to worry about in response. Think of times when you have found yourself worrying about fairly trivial things and ask whether you might have been feeling anxious to begin with.

Worry can also be an unhelpful cognitive approach to processing memories of events that have already happened. This process is often referred to as **rumination**. This involves thinking out alternative outcomes to the one that has actually happened. "If only I had (said/done...), things would have worked out differently." Again, some people believe that this amounts to learning from mistakes. However, most often it amounts to nothing more than mentally beating themselves up.

Stress is always a *physical* response to an immediate situation (which may be real or imaginary). As such, stress always concerns the present situation. But stress is always a positive... No, really!! Stress is your body's way of preparing itself to deal with a harmful or threatening situation. If you accept it as such, rather than seeking quick-fixes to try to escape from how your stress response makes you feel, you can begin to use your stress in a positive way.

STRESS DOESN'T KILL...
UNLESS YOU THINK IT DOES!

We have known for centuries that it is not events that trouble us, but the way we respond to them. This proposition was made as early as the 5th Century by Epictetus, and is a foundational idea behind the currently popular Cognitive Behavioural Therapy. More recently, however, scientists have discovered that the way we respond to stress can quite literally make the difference between life and death. In a 2012 study, Keller et al[*] sought to examine the whether the amount of stress and the perception of stress had an impact on mortality. After tracking more than 30,000 people for eight years, the study showed that people who experienced a large amount of stress *and* perceived stress to be harmful were 43 percent more likely to die prematurely than those who experienced less stress or – crucially – those who experienced a large amount of stress *but did not perceive stress to be a problem.*

According to Health Psychologist Kelly McGonigal[†] these findings suggest that 182,000 Americans die prematurely not as a result of stress itself, but because of the *belief* that stress is harmful. This would make stress the 15th biggest killer in the USA:

---

[*]   Keller, A., Litzelman, K., Wisk, L. E., Maddox, T., Cheng, E. R., Creswell, P. D., & Witt, W. P. (2012). *Does the perception that stress affects health matter? The association with health and mortality.* Health psychology: official journal of the Division of Health Psychology, American Psychological Association, 31(5), 677–684. doi:10.1037/a0026743

[†] Kelly McGonigal: *How to make stress your friend.* 2013 Ted Talk - http://youtu.be/RcGyVTAoXEU

1. Heart Disease (596,339)

2. Cancers (575,313)

3. Lung disease (143,382)

4. Stroke (128,931)

5. Accidents (122,777)

6. Alzheimer's disease (84,691)

7. Diabetes (73,282)

8. Flu (53,667)

9. Nephritis (45,731)

10. Suicide (38,285)

11. Septicaemia(35,539)

12. Liver disease (33,539)

13. Hypertension (27,477)

14. Parkinson's disease (23,107)

15. *Beliefs about stress (20,231)*

16. Pneumonitis (18,090)

Of course, this is mischievous because stress itself is not the killer. Most of these premature deaths will have been included in the figures for the other leading causes of death like heart disease, cancers and stroke. Nevertheless, the point is clear. If you believe that stress is harmful and to be avoided, then stress – and your response to it – will significantly lower your life expectancy.

Of course, the power of belief in relation to health has been known about for centuries. The *placebo* effect is so well understood that no scientist would accept the results of a clinical trial unless it included a control group who were given a placebo (dummy treatment) instead of the active treatment being studied. This is because even giving someone a sugar pill can have a positive effect on their health. Indeed, even when you tell someone you are giving them a sugar pill, their health still improves. And not all placebos are equal. Dummy injections are more effective than dummy pills, and red pills are more effective than blue pills.

The "placebo effect" works by encouraging the body's natural healing mechanisms to fight off illness. But what is going on with stress? It seems that our beliefs about stress have a direct impact on our cardiovascular system. The differences are subtle but important. A key part of the stress response is to pump extra blood to the muscles and to those areas of the brain involved in fight or flight. However, the way in which your body does this will depend upon your perception of stress. All of us will experience the pounding heart and rapid, shallow breathing that goes with the stress response. However, people who do not perceive stress to be harmful tend to have a coherent heartbeat whereas those who view stress as harmful have an erratic heartbeat. Also, those who perceive stress as harmful tend to have constricted blood vessels (which raises blood pressure) while those who do not view stress as a threat continue to have dilated blood vessels (allowing a fast circulation without raising blood pressure).

These differences help us understand one of the key debates within the field of stress management. We have been told that "some stress is good for you". This has led to a one-dimensional continuum view of stress:

Performance

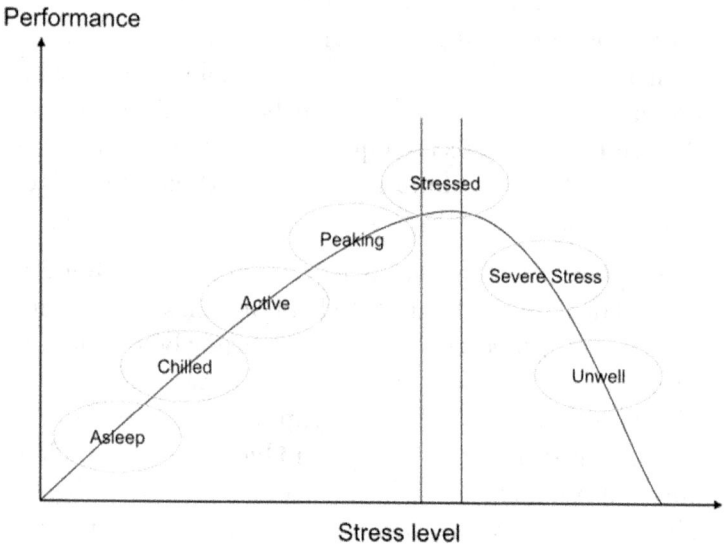

Stress level

However, the rate at which your stress response is running turns out to be much less important than the way you feel about it. If we create a matrix for high and low stress response and positive and negative feelings, a more rounded picture emerges:

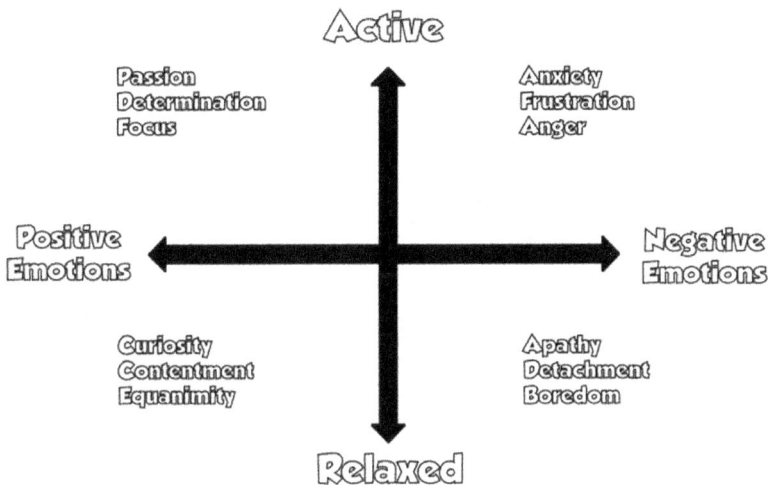

Active

Passion
Determination
Focus

Anxiety
Frustration
Anger

Positive Emotions

Negative Emotions

Curiosity
Contentment
Equanimity

Apathy
Detachment
Boredom

Relaxed

In this view of stress, both too much and not enough stress can be both a good and a bad thing depending upon how we *feel* about stress. A high degree of stress can produce dangerous feelings of anxiety, anger and frustration. But a low degree of stress may produce equally dangerous feelings of apathy, boredom and depression. On the other hand, a high degree of stress may produce positive feelings of passion, determination and focus, while a low degree of stress can produce feelings of contentment, equanimity and curiosity. The key determinant is not the stress response itself, but the way we engage emotionally with our stress.

Notice that the positive feelings associated with stress are those that sportspeople experience when they say they are "in the zone". They are the same as what some psychologists call "flow experiences". They are the same as the positive experiences that can come from meditation, yoga and tai chi. These experiences are often promoted using Mindfulness-Based Stress Reduction – something that began as a therapy, but has recently been adopted by business leaders, military personnel and politicians around the world.

EMERGENCY STRESS MANAGEMENT

Because traditional approaches to stress management have treated stress as an enemy to be overcome, most of the proposed solutions have involved finding ways of rapidly de-stressing. And while these have some short-term benefits, they are not really a long-term solution. You might, for example, learn some relaxation techniques or do some physical exercise. However, if the cause of your stress is ongoing, these are only really healthy replacements for less healthy quick-fixes like alcohol consumption or comfort eating.

It is important to remember that the human stress response is a product of thousands of years of evolution. Stress is not your enemy; it is a natural response to help you overcome unfavourable situations. And while an unconscious fight or flight response in modern circumstances is unlikely to be helpful, a more controlled use of stress can have positive results.

The mistake that most of us have been taught to make is to *avoid* stress or at least to avoid the sensation of stress. But this only results in a state of denial and/or the use of dangerous quick-fixes that ultimately cause illness. The more appropriate way to deal with stress is to learn to change it from a negative into a positive. The biggest barrier to this for most of us is that one of the first parts of the stress response is the shutting down of the part of the brain that process rational thought. Worse still, once this part of the brain - the neo prefrontal cortex - has shut down, we become unconscious of the fact that it has happened. So we tend to act from habit, and then *invent* rational explanations for our actions later on. This is why, for example, some people experience uncontrollable road rage when stuck in traffic. The rational understanding that we are all stuck in traffic is replaced with the irrational rage at the person in the vehicle immediately in front.

So the first thing we have to learn to do is to become mindful of how it feels when we begin to become stressed. Unfortunately, this cannot be done cognitively or even by getting in touch with our feelings. Rather, we need to get in touch with the raw emotion that connects how we are physically to what we feel (which in turn affects what we think and do). One reason why many people find practices like meditation, yoga and tai chi helpful is precisely because they consciously connect our physical, emotional and mental selves. It is also one reason why physical activity of any kind is helpful to managing stress.

The more self-aware we become, the better we get at noticing our stress response switching on when faced with a stressful situation. You may notice that your palms begin to sweat, or that your heart rate has increased, or that your breathing has become shallower and faster. It is at this point of self-awareness that you can act to switch from an unconscious and potentially harmful stress response to a conscious and potentially beneficial one.

Emergency stress management revolves around your breathing. This is the point where automatic physical processes meet those processes that can be consciously altered. It is impossible to consciously change the way your liver, kidneys, pancreas and even (directly) your heart operate. However, you are able to move your limbs and (to some extent) exercise control over your bowel and bladder. But your breathing is both unconscious (most of the time) and conscious (occasionally).

Provided that you can maintain conscious awareness, you will find that it is possible to focus your awareness. For example, you may have had a "bump in the night" experience. You might have been lying in bed, half asleep, when you hear an unfamiliar noise. Or you might have been walking in the dark and had the sensation of being followed. Immediately your awareness becomes more focused as your senses are directed to gathering more information about this potential threat. Your eyes search the darkness for the shape of a potential assailant, your ears strain to isolate unfamiliar sounds from the general background hum. It is this state of conscious, focussed attention that we need to employ when faced with modern stressors. However, the focus is not external. We need to focus our attention on our breathing. When we choose, we can alter the way we breathe. And this, in turn, allows us to change the way we feel. In a negative way, forcing yourself to breathe deeply and rapidly can trigger a sense of anxiety and even panic. Indeed, this type of breathing is what people who have panic disorders tend to do in response to the onset of a panic attack, even though this is always counter-productive. In a positive way, yoga and meditation teachers will use a range of breathing techniques that can produce affects as varied as alertness, focus, relaxation and calm. However, while yoga breathing techniques are interesting to learn, and can be helpful with building long-term resilience, they are often too complicated for emergency stress management.

Faced with the onset of your stress response, the four essential elements of breathing that you need to focus your attention on are to:

1. Breathe rhythmically - so long as you adopt a reasonably slow pace, it doesn't really matter what rhythm you choose. There are several breath pacing apps available, and a search on YouTube will bring up several breath pacing videos.

2. Breathe smoothly - allow the breath to come in and out in a single smooth motion. Avoid staccato breaths.

3. Maintain a comfortable air flow to avoid feeling short of breath or dizzy from too much air.

4. Focus your consciousness at the heart centre (the centre of your breast bone) - this is the best way of connecting with your feelings and the raw emotion that gives rise to them. Do not try to change the way you feel. Simply be aware of (but don't act on) how you are.

This technique will allow you to be active and alert (breathing coherently and maintaining dilated blood vessels) without slipping into the negative, unconscious side of stress. As such, it will help you to deal with the causes of your stress in a more appropriate manner. However, while this will move you away from the negative side of stress, it will not be sufficient to move you over to a more positive form of stress. For this, you will need to work on your personal resilience and develop a more positive focus in your life.

SHORT-TERM STRESS RELIEF

It is important to develop one or two quick and easy stress relief techniques that can be used as an alternative to the damaging quick-fixes that we unconsciously turn to in times of stress.

As we have seen, the benefits of substances like alcohol and sugar or behaviours like comfort eating and gambling is that they give more or less instant relief from the negative sensations of stress. However, instant relief comes at the expense of long-term health and wellbeing. And – as millions of smokers and dieters can attest – simply saying that you are going to quit is rarely a recipe for success.

In order to break a habitual quick fix, you must substitute it with an alternative. And since the aim is to quickly de-stress, this alternative must be quick and easy to access. The important thing is to choose one or two techniques and practice them regularly and systematically. You cannot expect them to work for you if you wait until you are stressed-out before trying them. If, for example, your quick fix is to have a glass of wine to unwind, then this has probably become second nature to you. You reach for a glass of wine after work without really thinking about it. And – crucially – you do so even if you are not stressed. So, if you are going to substitute an alternative, such as going for a walk, you need to make this a habit; doing it at the same time and for the same duration every day. That way, when you become stressed in future, you will be more likely to use walking as a de-stress technique than to revert to alcohol.

Building your armoury of healthy short-term stress relief techniques is important. However, these techniques are aimed primarily at avoiding unhealthy quick-fixes. They are not, in and of themselves, a means of developing your resilience to negative stress. Nor are they a means to harnessing and using positive stress.

In the appendix at the end of this guide, I have included a list of 30 rapid stress relief techniques that you can try.

RELAXATION

Unfortunately, traditional stress management teaches us that we have just two states of being – stressed and not stressed. The result of this erroneous view of stress is that far too many of us believe that any human experience that does not feel stressful must count as relaxation. So people believe that mundane activities like watching TV, listening to the radio, reading a book or just chatting with friends count as relaxation.

Of course, these things *can* sometimes bring about a superficial form of relaxation. However, they usually result in a whole range of feelings, some of which will be activating and stressful.

Recently, neurobiologists have discovered a human relaxation response that is opposite and equal to the stress response. This is not a state that most people experience in the course of our mundane day-to-day activities. Rather, it is a state that must be actively engaged through practices such as meditation, yoga, mindfulness and chanting. Moreover, it is a response that becomes accessible with practice.

The Relaxation Response

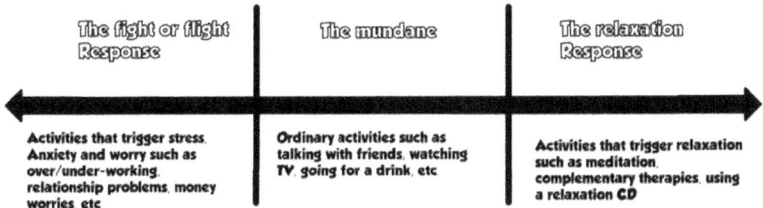

The fight or flight Response	The mundane	The relaxation Response
Activities that trigger stress, Anxiety and worry such as over/under-working, relationship problems, money worries, etc	Ordinary activities such as talking with friends, watching TV, going for a drink, etc	Activities that trigger relaxation such as meditation, complementary therapies, using a relaxation CD

The breathing technique for emergency stress management is a useful starting point for relaxation. However, the aim is not simply to avoid negative stress, but to move toward a state of physical, emotional and mental relaxation. Perhaps the easiest practice for achieving this is a process known as "body scan" relaxation (or meditation). A YouTube search will bring up pages of free video/audio guided relaxations that use this technique.

Body scan relaxation begins by becoming aware of your breathing. It involves becoming interested in and noticing the various sensations of your breath. How the air feels as it passes in and out of your nose, throat and chest. Is it warm or cool? Does it fill your whole lung? Is it fast or slow?

As you become interested in your breathing, so you begin to let go of your thoughts, worries and anxieties.

From here, a body scan relaxation involves focusing on the various parts of the body and relaxing and softening each in turn.

Relaxation really is as simple as that. However, most people struggle to achieve it because they only ever *try* to relax when they are particularly stressed. But this is a little like expecting to be able to play a musical instrument or succeed in a sport without putting in the practice. And when relaxation fails to materialise, all too many among us reach for the familiar quick-fixes – a bar of chocolate, large glass of wine or a cigarette – to try to de-stress.

For the best results, relaxation has to be practiced regularly. Preferably, this should be at the same time and in the same place every day. Initially, relaxation practice does not need to take much time. Indeed, few people can go more than about five minutes without fidgeting and letting their minds wander. So it is only with regular practice that you can develop deeper and longer relaxation.

The benefits of this, beyond removing the sensations associated with stress, are slower, more focused thinking and calmer emotions. These, in turn, allow you to navigate life with more clarity and purpose.

RESILIENCE

Just as stress enabled our ancestors to survive danger in prehistoric times, so stress can help us to survive and thrive in the modern world. But first we need to build personal resilience so that our stress response operates in a healthy manner and does not run out of control.

The key to shifting from being the victim of your stress to mastering it is the development of personal resilience at every level of your being:

Physical wellbeing

A negative response to stress can take a toll on your physical health. It can have direct effects on your body (such as raising your blood pressure, increasing fat deposits around vital organs, causing digestive problems, straining your heart, etc). It affects your body indirectly because of the unhealthy quick-fix things you do to de-stress (such as smoking, drinking too much alcohol, comfort eating, etc). While your body can cope with this in the short-term, you will become ill if you have to cope with high levels of stress for prolonged periods.

To avoid becoming unwell, it is important for you to address the physical consequences of stress in healthy ways. This means giving up smoking and cutting down on alcohol, caffeine, chocolate and other fatty and sugary foods. It also means adopting healthy approaches to:

o   Breathing

o   Posture

o   Activity

o   Sleep and relaxation

o   Diet

In the longer term, making healthy lifestyle choices in each of these areas will improve your resilience to stress as well as improving your general wellbeing.

Breathing

As we have seen, a simple breathing technique is all that you need to avoid negative stress. Simply breathing gently, rhythmically and smoothly using the whole of your lungs and with a focus at the centre of your chest will rapidly cause your heart rate to become coherent. This, in turn, will allow you to maintain a positive mental focus. However, although this sounds fairly straightforward, there are strong forces working against you. When you get stressed, it only takes a moment for the blood supply to switch from the neo prefrontal cortex (the bit of your brain that does the thinking) to the much older reptile brain (the bit that runs your habits). Once this happens, you will fall into habitual (quick-fix) behaviours, and your body will respond as if you had come face to face with a large, hungry predator. Your breathing will become fast and shallow, your heart rate will rise and become erratic, and your blood vessels will constrict. It will take time before your system calms again and you can start getting back to normal.

So the trick is to pre-empt this negative stress response by consciously deploying your breathing technique *before* your system goes into habit mode. In part, this means learning to identify how your system operates so that you become much more mindful of your stress response. In part, however, it involves practicing breathing techniques on a regular basis so that your body becomes used to breathing in these ways.

You may want to explore the many breathing techniques used in yoga, or you may just want to practice a single relaxation breathing technique every day. Whether you go to a class, use one of the many YouTube videos, or purchase a relaxation CD, the important thing is to practice until it becomes second nature.

Posture

One physical response to stress is for your body to curl in on itself. We evolved to do this in order to coil our muscles (ready to fight or flee) and to protect the vital organs in the chest and abdomen.

While adopting a crouched posture isn't too much of a problem in the short-term, in time it will have a negative impact on your health and wellbeing. You will experience aches and pains in your back, shoulders, neck and head as a result of the tension in the muscles. Your breathing will be impaired by the additional pressure on your lungs and diaphragm. The pressure on your abdomen will also impact on the way your vital organs function.

More subtly, the way you see and interact with the world will change. To appreciate this, try deliberately exaggerating the posture by hunching your shoulders and neck forward. Without changing position, check your field of vision. Now exaggerate an open posture with your back straight, shoulders back and head upright. Check your field of vision again. See the difference?

Taking time regularly to re-adjust your posture and to gently stretch your body can be helpful. If you want to do more, exercise programmes such as Alexander Technique, Pilates and Yoga are particularly helpful for correcting poor posture.

Activity

Stress can leave you feeling exhausted and just wanting to lie down or sit in front of the TV. While this is okay in the short-term, it can become a habit. And the less you do, the less you are able to do.

Your fight or flight mechanism evolved to help your body move quickly in response to a threat. So being physically active can help counteract the effects of stress directly. Being physically active is also an essential part of healthy living, and will help you become more resilient in the face of stress in the longer term. Ideally you should try to do something physical to the point that it increases your heart and breathing rate for about 30 minutes a day on most days.

Being physically active need not involve joining a gym or buying expensive sports equipment (although this is fine if you can commit to it). Just taking a half-hour walk at lunch time, doing some gardening, or tidying around the house counts as physical activity.

If you can engage in activities you enjoy and especially where there is a social element (e.g., going swimming or cycling with a friend) you are much more likely to keep doing them – and make them a habit!

Sleep and relaxation

Sleep and relaxation are directly affected by anger, anxiety and worry. This is because your stress response will activate in response to thoughts and feelings *about* an imagined threat in exactly the same way as it does when faced with a real threat. So, for example, worrying about the (imagined) presentation you have to give tomorrow will make you as stressed as you would be while giving the (actual) presentation. The difference is that when you actually give the presentation, you will deploy your stress response positively, for example using your extra alertness to recall facts about your subject, or even to throw in some jokes to help build rapport with your audience.

But lying in bed allowing your mind to conjure up imaginary stressors is entirely negative. And the more angry, anxious or worried you get in response to these phantoms, the harder it is to relax or to get a good night's sleep. Over time your lack of sleep (and the resulting tiredness) will leave you even more susceptible to anger, anxiety and worry. Also, prolonged sleep problems have been linked to mental illnesses such as anxiety disorders and depression and physical illnesses like dementia and diabetes.

There are many things you can do to improve your sleep and relaxation (the Life Surfing booklet *Getting to Sleep* goes into greater detail on this topic). As a starting point, you should avoid substances and activities that overstimulate you (such as coffee, computer games and excess alcohol) in the run up to bedtime. Instead, try to do things that promote sleep and relaxation (such as taking a warm bath, having a milky drink or listening to a relaxation CD). It helps to get into a routine. Try to take 15-20 minutes every day to relax. Find somewhere quiet and comfortable where you won't be disturbed. Try to use the same time and place every day. Similarly with sleep, try to go to bed at the same time every night. Keep the bedroom free of clutter, and avoid having computers, TVs, phones and (if possible) clocks in the bedroom.

It is important not to try to "catch up" on sleep during the day. This will just leave you unable to sleep at night. Also, try to avoid lying in on the weekend, as this can also disrupt your sleep routine.

If sleep and relaxation are particularly difficult for you, you may want to think about trying a complementary therapy like aromatherapy, massage or reflexology. Alternatively, you could join a local relaxation, tai chi or yoga class.

Diet

There are several ways in which stress can affect your diet. Most directly, substances such as alcohol, caffeine, chocolate and sugar contain chemicals that provide short-term relief from the effects of adrenaline. You may find that you unconsciously reach for food and drink that contain these substances when you are stressed.

Psychologically, you may be inclined to comfort eat as a way of feeling better when you are stressed. You may "treat yourself" to a big bar of chocolate, a pack of cream cakes or a tub of ice cream—this is okay once in a while, but it will affect your weight and your general sense of wellbeing if it becomes a habit. And too much sugar in your diet will increase your risk of developing a range of serious physical illnesses such as cancers, diabetes, heart disease and liver disease.

Prolonged stress can deaden your senses of smell and taste (this becomes particularly pronounced in people who develop depression). One result of this is that you may begin to choose foods that are heavily flavoured, salty or sweet. In most cases, these foods will be unhealthy and will have a negative impact on your wellbeing in the longer-term. You may also be tempted to opt for foods (simple carbohydrates like sugar and sweets) that give a quick energy burst by increasing your blood sugar levels. However, the energy burst will be short lived, and you will quickly feel tired again. The alternative is to opt for complex carbohydrates (like potatoes, pasta and rice) that increase your energy levels more slowly, but maintain your energy levels for much longer.

There is a range of foods that are thought to improve mood and energy levels (you can find out more in the Life Surfing Booklet *Food & Mood*). However, perhaps more important is learning to eat a balanced diet that is low in fat and high in fibre, with plenty of fruit, pulses and vegetables.

Emotional Wellbeing

Stress is not just about external events. It is also to do with the way you respond.

One of the dangers facing you as you become more stressed is that you turn emotions such as guilt, anger, self-blame and hate in upon yourself. This will impact badly on the way you think and behave.

Learning to manage and express your feelings in a healthy way will help you to improve your resilience to stressors in the longer-term.

The most important thing you can do is talk about your feelings. This doesn't mean opening up to anyone irrespective of whether they want to hear about your feelings. Rather, it means finding a trusted friend or relative who will give you the time and space to express how you are feeling.

In the absence of someone close enough to you for you to feel comfortable about expressing your feelings, there are several alternatives:

o   Use a helpline such as Community Advice and Listening Line, Saneline or Samaritans. If you are in employment, your employer may operate a telephone counselling service. You may also have access to telephone counselling if you have medical insurance.

o   See if you can access face-to-face counselling. There may be a counsellor based at your local doctors' surgery (although there will most probably be a waiting list). Alternatively, there are many charities that offer counselling. If you have sufficient income, you may want to pay for private counselling—but be aware that the costs can mount up.

o   Use online social media to interact with people who have similar issues to you.

You might also want to think about engaging in creative activities that may help you express your feelings less directly. Arts, crafts, music and poetry are all ways in which people can express themselves.

Mental Wellbeing

The more stressed you become, the more likely you are to develop irrational, unrealistic and often negative thoughts and beliefs. Unfortunately, this is an insidious process that prevents you noticing what is happening.

Unpicking thoughts and beliefs can be difficult to do on your own. This is why it can be helpful to seek counselling or a psychological therapy such as Cognitive Behavioural Therapy (CBT), which can help you develop a more realistic appraisal of your thoughts and beliefs.

If you are unable to access face-to-face therapy, there is a computerised programme called *Beating the Blues* that is available through the NHS. There are also several online CBT programmes that can be accessed free of charge.

Social engagement

Prolonged negative stress will often affect your ability to function socially. It impairs your concentration, memory and motor functions which in turn affect your performance at work. It also leaves you tired, making you less likely to engage socially and more likely to withdraw into your home or even under your duvet.

Unfortunately, withdrawal makes you even more susceptible to negative stress. So it is easy to get into a vicious downward spiral.

The only way of reversing this is to engage socially even if you don't feel like it. The important thing is to use the increased arousal that comes with stress to help you focus your engagement on those social activities that leave you feeling positive. This can be difficult because we have learned to put up with and accept social circumstances that we find negative simply because "they are expected of us". For example, every morning around the world, millions of people have the negative experience of getting up early to travel to a job that they hate doing. They do it in part because they have to – they need the money. But they also do it out of misplaced loyalty, a desire to please other people, and a need to avoid being seen as feckless were they to stop doing it. Of course, millions of other people look forward to the coming day because the work they do challenges them, bolsters their self-esteem, and leaves them feeling positive.

Similar examples can be given for romantic relationships, peer group relationships and neighbourhood relationships. As with employment, these can all be negative, positive, or simply mundane. However, if you experience negative stress as a result of engaging with them, rather than treating this as an illness to be cured or treated, look on it as a warning sign that things are not as they should be. Then use the energy that your stress response provides to focus properly on making the changes required to start living the life you deserve.

THE CANARY IN THE MINE

Poisonous gases trapped deep within rock formations have always presented a threat to miners. Today a range of technologies is used to detect and mitigate this risk. However, in years gone by the only way miners could detect the presence of toxic gas was to take a small bird in a cage into the mine with them. Because a small bird has smaller lungs, and because it breathes very rapidly, it will succumb to the effects of poison gas before the miners. So, when the canary stopped singing, the miners would run!

Stress in the modern world functions in the same way. Whether you notice the stress response itself, the feelings it leaves you with, or the behaviours (drinking, smoking, withdrawal, etc) you adopt, it is a wakeup call telling you that something is wrong.

The problem is that we have been encouraged to think about negative stress as an illness to be cured. Indeed, there is confusion about where "stress" ends and mental illnesses like anxiety and depression begin. This is not helped by far too many people using the word "stress" as a euphemism for these more stigmatised conditions. So when someone begins to feel the negative effects of prolonged stress, they are inclined (and encouraged) to see a doctor and seek *treatment*.

Unfortunately, the medical profession does not take someone's social circumstances into account when making a diagnosis. So, for example, you may go to a doctor with the fallout from prolonged negative stress that is the result of a relationship breakdown or too much pressure/bullying at work, and all the doctor is interested in is treating your symptoms:

- o You can't sleep?.. We have a pill for that!

- o Your heart rate is too fast?.. We have a pill for that!

- o You feel unhappy all the time?.. We have a pill for that!

Psychologist Abraham Maslow came up with the "law of instrument". Put simply, "if the only tool you have is a hammer, then every problem starts to look like a nail". Because doctors only have pills, when you visit them with stress-related symptoms, they tend to see a chemical imbalance. Similarly, because counsellors and therapists deal in thoughts and feelings, they tend to see a package of inappropriate mental and emotional responses. And while both therapy and pills may have their place, they tend not to address the underlying issues that gave rise to the problem in the first place. This would be the mining equivalent of trying to teach miners to breathe poisonous gases!

Rather than encouraging you to take a pill, your awareness of negative stress is telling you to take *Action!!*

WORK, MONEY AND MOTIVATION

The experience of negative stress and its fallout opens the way to ask some searching questions about the situation you are in. And, ultimately, there are only two things that you can do:

o   Change the situation

o   Change the way you respond to the situation.

For example, someone who has road rage could choose an anger management route. They could learn to understand their thoughts, beliefs and feelings and practice techniques to change these in a more positive direction. Rather than seeing the times they are stuck in traffic as periods of frustration in which other people are in their way, they could see them as a space that they can use for themselves; perhaps listening to their favourite music or an audio book as an alternative to getting wound up. Alternatively, they could adopt a far more radical approach by questioning why they are in a car stuck in traffic in the first place. Many people are only in their cars in traffic because they think they need to commute to a job they hate in order to pay their bills. And while many can benefit by changing the way they respond, some will simply opt to change the situation. Often, the costs of owning and running a car (or using public transport) can run to several thousand pounds a year. So one option is to simply drop out of the rat race – take a cut in pay in order to get work within walking or cycling distance to home and your living standard can be maintained.

Whether you choose to change your situation or learn to manage how you respond to it will largely depend on the underlying assumptions and beliefs you have about the world and your place within it. These are what motivate us to do anything. But they are often unconscious and as much to do with stories we were told as children. For example, in the 1950s you were guaranteed a decent, well-paid job if you studied hard, passed your exams and graduated from university. Today, many youngsters continue to believe this story to the extent that they take on tens of thousands of pounds of debt which will have the perverse effect of preventing them doing the middle tier jobs that 1950s graduates used to take to springboard their careers. If you have large student debts and you want to have a family and a home of your own, you have to compete for high paying jobs mostly in the banking and finance sector, irrespective of whether this is what you want to do. The only alternative for many graduates is to work in a low paying job where income falls below the threshold for paying back the debt, and do this for long enough for the debt to be written off (assuming the UK government doesn't adopt the US policy of never forgiving student debt and never allowing students to declare bankruptcy). So while having a degree continues to give an advantage in the labour market, it is no longer the guarantee of success that it had once been. Indeed, alternatives such as modern apprenticeships and in-work training can often be at least as good for career building as a university education.

We have told ourselves similar stories about the value of hard work. Certainly in the 1950s and 60s it was possible to secure a good standard of living for a job in industry or construction; particularly if you could get an apprenticeship. However, some of the hardest workers in modern Britain have such low incomes that they have to draw tax credits and housing benefit to make ends meet.

But perhaps the most damaging story we tell ourselves is that money is the answer to our problems. We find this in the narrative about "work-life balance" which is supposed to give us a stress-free life. The very concept of work-life balance takes as its implicit starting point the view that there are two separate entities – or work and our lives. By definition in this concept, work is something outside and alien to life. It is something that you just have to suck up in order to obtain the money you need to finance your life. So the concept of work-life balance assumes that obtaining money is such an important goal that we should engage in activities considered alien to life simply to obtain it.

In recent years, attempts to develop measures of national wellbeing and happiness have helped to give the lie to the idea that money is an important goal. Actually, something more subtle is going on. It turns out that money is an issue where standards of living are low. However, once you reach a point where money can be taken off the table – where a decent standard of living is reached – additional money does not produce additional happiness.

So insofar as money is a goal, the aim is to have *enough* rather than to keep accumulating. And this seems to be borne out in health outcomes too. For while poverty is a major public health problem, so too is extreme inequality. And not just for the poor. The richest people in the UK and USA have lower life expectancies than the upper classes in less unequal European and Scandinavian countries.

It gets worse. It turns out that money is the enemy of creativity and productivity. According to most economists, a system of sanctions and rewards is the best way to motivate people. Like so much in economics, nobody actually researched this, they just assumed that because it sounds plausible, it must be correct (just as they assumed that we had reached "the great moderation" of the global economy in 2008). But when psychologists conducted experiments to prove this, they found something much more interesting is happening.

When work is mechanistic, mechanical and unthinking, a system of rewards and sanctions does indeed increase productivity. So, for example, paying 1970s production line workers additional bonuses for speeding up the line helped to increase production. However, once the work involved thinking and creativity (as is the case in the majority of modern employment) paying additional money resulted in *decreased* productivity. Once again, it became clear that money is only an issue where workers do not enjoy a decent standard of living. But

---

* Dan Ariely, Uri Gneezy, George Loewenstein, and Nina Mazar. *Large Stakes and Big Mistakes.* 2005. Federal Reserve Bank of Boston

once you reach the point that money is no longer a concern, then rewards such as bonus schemes actually harm productivity – one reason why governments and shareholders should seriously reassess the bonus systems used in the finance industry.

So, many of the stories that we learned about how the world ought to be and what we should be doing within it, turn out to be myths. This understanding paves the way both to change how you think and feel about your situation or whether to change the situation itself.

One of the best starting points for considering how to respond to the circumstances that are responsible for your negative stress is to consider whether the things you are doing today are the most important things in life. One way of thinking about this is to look at the things that people value or regret on their deathbeds. In her book, *Top 5 Regrets of the Dying*, Bronnie Ware, a palliative care nurse who spent years caring for dying patients, sets out the five main regrets of dying people:

- o Not having the courage to be true to yourself (living your life to other people's standards and expectations)

- o Working too hard/long (missing time with your partner and children)

- o Not expressing your feelings

- o Losing touch with friends

- o Not allowing yourself to be happy.

All five regrets relate to living a life to please others – employers, family members, neighbours or "public expectations" – or refusing to take the risks required to lead the life you want. Sadly, only at the time of death do many people realise that these were choices that had been available to them.

In many cases, your negative stress is a warning that the life you are living is not the life you wanted for yourself. As such, there are choices that will have to be made. Only you can make these choices. But you may find that you want to work with a coach, counsellor or therapist to help you work out what is best for you.

AUTONOMY, MASTERY AND PURPOSE

If money, hard work and pleasing others fail to motivate us, what does?

According to behavioural economist Daniel Pink[*], once people have enough income for money not to be an issue, motivation has three dimensions:

o Autonomy

o Mastery

o Purpose.

In a workplace setting, autonomy means giving people the space to get on with their work unhindered. But it can also mean allowing people to experiment with ideas that are not directly to do with their work. For example, tech firms like Google allow employees to work on projects of their own for up to 20 percent of their time in work. It is this activity – apparently unrelated to work – that produces many of the best technological developments. A desire for autonomy is also a reason why millions of people have turned to self-employment or have set up their own businesses, even though this almost always means taking a cut in income – at least to begin with.

Autonomy is also important outside work. However, in this arena, autonomy is often more to do with not living life according to what you think others want. That is, learning to be true to yourself. This is more than simply doing what you please. And it is not about being selfish

---

[*] Daniel H. Pink. 2011. *Drive: The Surprising Truth About What Motivates Us.* Penguin Books.

– we are social beings, and autonomy has its boundaries. Rather, it is about recognising that each one of us has skills and abilities that have to be nurtured and developed. We need to align the rest of our lives with these if we are to get the most out of life.

This takes us to a central part of what motivates us – the desire for self-mastery. The two most obvious popular arenas for observing the quest for self-mastery are in music and sport. Both require some raw talent and aptitude. However, all else is practice. To become a concert musician or a national or international athlete requires at least 10,000 hours of practice. Why would anyone do this? Certainly not for the money! The key reason why musicians and sportspeople practice is because it produces an almost mystical state of being that psychologists call a "flow experience". More colloquially, sportspeople talk about "being in the zone". In this state, athletes and musicians find that their performance appears to become effortless, and this in turn creates a profound sense of satisfaction.

It isn't only athletes and musicians who enjoy these flow experiences. It turns out that anyone who is engaged in an activity that they deeply enjoy, and that requires a degree of skill and practice can also have flow experiences. And, these flow experiences have many overlaps with the stress response – they involve focus, a narrowing of the senses, elevated heart and breathing rates. However, they differ from the negative stress response because they involve positive emotions such as passion and determination.

Unfortunately, there is a problem with flow experiences – you cannot reproduce them continuously at the same level of skill. That is, as you become used to performing at a particular level of self-mastery, so the number and depth of flow experiences subside. The only way to maintain these flow experiences is to constantly improve your skill levels. But to do this in the long-term requires a purpose that goes beyond the activity itself. This is why so many amateurs quit or get stuck at an intermediate skill level.

Remember when you first learned to drive. You probably fumbled around quite a bit. Everything took time because you had to think consciously about what you were doing. In addition to focusing your senses on what was happening around you, you had to coordinate unfamiliar motor skills (selecting gears, depressing and lifting foot pedals, switching lights and indicators on and off, etc). Gradually, you developed mastery over driving. You began to be able to focus your senses on important things (other traffic, pedestrians, potential hazards), while your motor skills became habits, allowing you to control your vehicle without needing to think about it. You may even have developed flow experiences when driving during this early phase of mastery.

Notice that driving is always "stressful" – it would be dangerous to drive in a completely relaxed state. Indeed, it is illegal to drive under the influence of substances like alcohol or cannabis that artificially induce a relaxed state. The stress you experienced when learning was most probably negative. You may have felt anxious, and physical sensations such as a racing heart and rapid breathing may have made the experience of driving unpleasant. However, as you developed your driving skills, your stress tended to manifest positively as focus and determination. You had begun to use your stress response properly – as a natural physical process that helps you succeed in a difficult situation.

But driving – and other skills – cannot produce positive stress and flow experiences indefinitely. The more habitual the practice becomes, the more we take it for granted. It becomes mundane, and can only become stressful again if additional challenges are undertaken. For example, a driver may choose to learn advanced driving or even take up track racing in order to further develop their skills and to challenge themselves further.

Of course, most people who learn to drive do not do so primarily to develop driving mastery. Most simply want a driving licence so that they can commute to work, do their weekly shop, and ferry the kids around. This gives a hint of the final element of positive stress – *purpose*.

The whole gamut of human activities offers the possibility of stress, challenge and mastery. Whether it is learning to drive, playing a musical instrument, developing computer skills, doing arts and crafts or writing and publishing a book, we can develop so long as we have purpose. However, for most of us, the purposes of these kinds of activity are secondary – they are a means to an end rather than an end in themselves. So although they provide a challenge that produces initial negative stress followed by positive stress in the form of focus and determination, they tend not to result in flow experiences (at least not to any depth or duration).

There is an old saying that "if you do something you love, you will never have to work again". This alludes to the idea that each of us has a more profound purpose to our lives. This will be something that so aligns our physical, emotional and mental being that it feels like second nature. The idea that each life has intrinsic purpose is common around the world in both religious and secular discourse. In Eastern traditions, this sense of life purpose is known as "Dharma". In Western Christianity, it is known as "Mission". In a more secular expression, educationalist Sir Ken Robinson has talked about being *in your element*[†]:

> "The Element is where natural aptitude meets personal passion. To begin with it means that you are doing something for which you have a natural feel... But being in your Element is more than doing things you are good at. Many people are good at things they don't really care for. To be in your Element you have to love it too."

From this perspective, the experience of negative stress is almost always the result of a misalignment between your Element and the circumstances you find yourself in. This requires action to bring your circumstances into line with this deeper life purpose. This may mean – as we saw with driving – learning and developing mastery over the various skills required to succeed. However, it

---

[†] Robinson, K. 2013. *Finding your Element: How to discover your talents and passions and transform your life.* Penguin Books.

may be that you are in the wrong situation (relationship, job, neighbourhood, etc). If this is the case, only changing the situation will serve to overcome negative stress in the long-term.

So how do you find your Dharma/ Element/ Mission/ Purpose?

The three key questions to ask here are:

- o What are you good at?

- o What do you love?

- o Who do you care about?

These are easier asked than answered. But try to imagine a time in your life when everything seemed to be going just right. I don't mean just recall it. I mean really take yourself back to the experience. Try to remember the details. What were you wearing? Who else was there? What were they doing? What were you doing? How did you feel? What did you achieve?

These kinds of experiences can help us tease out the outline of our personal purpose. But they also point to some more negative questions:

- o What got in the way?

- o Why did you not develop your skills and abilities?

- o What external barriers have you faced?

- o What internal barriers did you erect?

All too often, we find ourselves doing things that we hate or don't enjoy because we feel pressured to fit in. People will stay in a poor or even abusive relationship because we fear the change that walking away will entail. People will stay in soul-destroying employment rather than seek the type of work we love, or embark on our new business ventures because we fear the loss of income and dislocation more than we anticipate success.

Change, of course, can feel threatening. It is risky, and it may create loss and heartache. But ultimately, so too does staying put in a situation that you hate. This risks the full range of negative emotions like resentment, jealousy, anger, intolerance, etc. But change can also be positive. It can unlock your passions and allow you to thrive. As the writer Mark Twain once observed:

> "Twenty years from now you will be more disappointed by the things that you didn't do than by the ones that you did do..."

TAKE ACTION NOW!

We have been taught to treat stress as an illness to be treated. However, stress is not, in and of itself, an illness. Indeed, it turns out that stress only seems to develop into illness for those people who view stress as a problem. That is, those who internalise the view that "stress *is* an illness" are most likely to get ill as a result. Those who experience high stress but do not view it as a problem or an illness have the same life expectancy as those with little or no stress.

The implication of seeing stress as an illness is that we have sought to provide treatments for it. We have seen a massive expansion in the numbers of people worldwide taking sedatives like *Valium* and antidepressants like *Prozac* to treat "stress-related" conditions like anxiety and depression. And while these treatments may be of some benefit, they are not an alternative to taking *action*!

Like the canary in the mine, the human stress response – when experienced as a negative – is a sign that all is not well. It is a sign that one's life and one's circumstances have become misaligned. In such circumstances, it is easy to give in to the fear of change, seeking instead, a means of continuing with things as they are while trying to feel differently about them. This is one reason why the promise of antidepressant drugs and cognitive behavioural therapy are so persuasive. Both appear to provide means to continue to live in unpleasant circumstances by helping us to feel better about our situation.

One statistic rarely mentioned in the medical literature is that within two years, people who take antidepressants or use CBT have the same outcomes as people who do not have these "treatments". The people who recover, it seems, are not those who treat their negative stress as illness, but those who use the energy of positive stress to change their circumstances. Of course, this process of change is difficult. But with hindsight, people often find that they had used far too much of their energy holding on to jobs, relationships and circumstances that had been making them ill. These people often regret that they did not use the energy of their stress in a positive manner to give them the drive, focus and passion to follow their dreams at an earlier point in their lives.

So the choice is yours. You can use the stress management techniques set out in this booklet just to provide temporary relief. Alternatively, you can begin to make longer-term lifestyle changes to move your life in a more positive and satisfying direction.

I don't promise you that change is easy. But I do promise you that one way or another, change is the only way of overcoming negative stress in the long-term.

APPENDIX: 30 FIVE-MINUTE STRESS RELIEF TECHNIQUES

1. **Sip green tea**. Green tea is a source of L-Theanine, a substance that helps relieve feelings of anger

2. **Tighten and relax your muscles**. Isolate each of the muscle groups in your body, beginning at your feet and working up to your head. Tighten and relax each muscle group in turn

3. **Eat some mango**. Mangoes are a source of a chemical called Linalool that helps to reduce stress levels

4. **Meditate**. Take 5 minutes to sit somewhere quite and clear your mind. The best way to do this is to find a focus, such as concentrating on the breath at the tip of your nose

5. **Run cold water on your wrist**. Cooling the major arteries that run through the wrist helps relieve stress

6. **Tidy up your clutter**. Clutter and mess add to feelings of stress. Clearing up and just leaving out the things you need can contribute to a sense of calm

7. **Eat something crunchy**. Chewing is one of the ways in which the body responds to stress. Eating something healthy like a stick of celery can help you de-stress without putting on the pounds

8. **Look out of the window**. Take some time just to sit and focus on your surroundings. Really notice the environment, people, nature, colours, sounds and smells

9. **Breathe**. Slow, smooth and rhythmic breathing using the whole of the lung can quickly reduce stress and help promote a sense of calm

10. **Dance**. Any form of cardio-vascular activity can help with stress. Because dancing requires being aware of your body, and moving in time with music, this also promotes a sense of calm

11. **Acupressure**. Acupressure is a touching therapy that can relieve stress and promote calm. It is best to see a therapist for acupressure, but you can try relaxing on an acupressure mat

12. **Slowly eat a square of chocolate**. Chocolate can help lower stress levels (although too much is bad for you). Try really concentrating on the smell, texture and taste of the chocolate as you slowly consume it

13. **Creative visualisation**. Visualise a situation in which you feel calm and positive about yourself, your surroundings and your life. This helps you break out of stress

14. **Walk or jog**. Cardio-vascular exercise helps to reduce stress, anxiety and depression. If you are able to do this outdoors, where you can get sunlight and fresh air, this will add to your sense of calm

15. **Count backwards from 100**. Counting backwards requires the same kind of focus used in meditation, and can quickly relieve stress

16. **Chew some gum**. Chewing is one of the ways in which the body responds to stress. Chewing a small amount of gum will help relieve stress, and it is a lot better than comfort eating as it avoids weight gain

17. **Squeeze a stress ball**. Like chewing, fist clenching is a natural response to stress. Using a stress ball to clench and relax your fist can help dissipate stress and anger

18. **Catch the sun**. Exposure to sunlight is known to lift your mood. Getting outdoors is particularly important to those working in the unnatural light of modern workplaces

19. **Write**. Writing down the things that are troubling you can help you put them into perspective. You can also write down anything that you need to remember later on—this will save you worrying about it for the rest of the day

20. **Eat some honey**. Honey is thought to contain substances that improve mood. It is also a healthier way of getting a sweet taste than using sugar or artificial sweeteners

21. **Laugh**. Laughter benefits us physically as the body has to breathe differently and blood flow

is increased. It is also good psychologically, taking our minds away from our worries. So take 5 minutes to watch a YouTube comedy clip or read a cartoon strip

22. **Brush your hair**. The repetitiveness of brushing and the physical sense of the brush massaging your scalp can help relieve stress and bring about a sense of calm

23. **Smell some citrus**. Citrus is thought to raise noradrenaline—a neurotransmitter associated with stress, anxiety and depression. Taking time to really focus on the scent of citrus fruit can help relieve stress

24. **Rest your head**. Taking 5 minutes to lie down comfortably and let go of your tension will help relieve stress—but be careful not to nod off!

25. **Create and use a Zen zone**. Find a calm space where you can go to take 5 minutes away from the hustle and bustle of life. This could be a corner of a local park or just a quiet part of the office

26. **Massage your foot on a ball**. You can get a quick (and cheap) alternative to a full reflexology massage by rolling your feet over a golf ball

27. **Stretch**. Muscle tension is one of the ways the body holds stress. Stretching can help loosen the muscles and relieve feelings of stress

28. **Close your eyes**. Closing your eyes can help break the link with your stressful surroundings

29. **Massage your hands**. This can be especially useful for people who use keyboards, people who drive, and people who work in manual jobs. Take 5 minutes to gently but firmly massage every part of both hands—focusing on the sensations

30. **Take time to be alone**. Taking 5 minutes away from other people can help you unwind and gather your thoughts.

IF YOU FOUND THIS BOOK HELPFUL, PLEASE RECOMMEND IT TO OTHERS!!

Thank you for reading *Good Stress - Bad Stress* I am sure you will find it useful both to you and to those who care about you.

If *Good Stress - Bad Stress* was helpful to you, it will also be helpful to others. So please take the time to leave a review, so that you can help to bring this book to their attention and help them too.

ALSO BY TIM WATKINS

○ *Beating Anxiety: A Guide to Managing and Overcoming Anxiety Disorders.* This Life Surfing guide explains what anxiety is, how it is treated, and - crucially - what steps you can take to help yourself recover and sustain your personal wellbeing.

○ *Depression: A guide to managing and overcoming depression.* This guide provides you with an introduction to what depression is, how it is treated, and - crucially - what you can do to help yourself overcome the condition and create long-term personal wellbeing.

○ *Depression Workbook: 70 Self-help techniques for recovering from depression.* This book provides you with 70 self-help techniques covering the seven key areas of your personal wellbeing.

○ *Distress to De-stress: Understanding and managing stress in everyday life.* This Life Surfing guide explains what stress is, and - crucially - what healthy steps you can take to manage stress and promote long-term personal wellbeing. The guide includes 30 stress management techniques.

○ *Food for Mood: A guide to healthy eating for mental health.* In this guide book, Tim Watkins explains how mental health problems can impact on diet and how you can improve your diet by using foods from the helpful lists of good mood foods set out in the guide. We also provide some good mood food starter recipes for anyone who is relatively new to cooking.

○ *Getting to sleep: A guide to overcoming stress-related sleep problem.* With 1 in 3 of us experiencing stress-related insomnia, this important Life Surfing guide will give you a good understanding of sleep and - crucially - the steps you can take to improve the quality and duration of your sleep... night after night.

○ *How to Help: A guide to helping someone manage mental distress.* In this Life Surfing guide, we explain what mental health and mental illness are, and - crucially - the steps that you can take to help someone experiencing mental health problems or mental illness.

○ *Helping Hands: How to Help Someone Else Cope with Mental Health Problems.* Worried about the wellbeing of a relative, friend, colleague or client? Not sure what to do or worried you might say or do the wrong thing? Helping Hands will provide you with an understanding of wellbeing, and knowledge of mental illness, and will show you how you can help and support someone who has, or is at risk of developing, a mental health problem. Helping Hands also sets out a great deal of what has been learned about self-help and self-management strategies for recovery from mental illness over the last 25 years.

○ *No More Panic - A Guide to overcoming panic attacks and recovering from panic disorder.* Half of us will experience a panic attack at some time in our lives. For those who do, the experience can be quite literally terrifying. For many the experience is so unpleasant that they avoid similar situations in future. Some develop disabling panic disorders and agoraphobia. In this book, we set out what we - and others - have learned about panic attacks, and how anyone can overcome them... permanently.

www.ingramcontent.com/pod-product-compliance
Lightning Source LLC
Chambersburg PA
CBHW050554280326
41933CB00011B/1840